Methylene Blue Guide

Exploring the Uses and Benefits of Methylene Blue

By

Gilroy Howie
Copyright@2023

Table of Contents

CHAPTER 1

Introduction to Methylene Blue

1.1 What is Methylene Blue?

Methylene Blue, often abbreviated as MB, is a synthetic dye and medication with a deep blue or greenish-blue color. It is chemically known as 3,7-bis(dimethylamino)phenothiazin-5-ium chloride. Methylene Blue belongs to the phenothiazine family of compounds and is characterized by its versatile properties and wide range of applications. Its distinctive color and unique chemical structure make it easily distinguishable, and it plays a crucial role in various fields, including medicine, biology, and environmental science.

The compound derives its name from its blue coloration and has a rich history dating back to the 19th century. Methylene Blue is a cationic dye, which means it carries a positive charge. This property makes it readily interact with negatively charged molecules, including various biological and cellular components, allowing it to be employed in a multitude of applications.

1.2 Historical Significance

The history of Methylene Blue is intertwined with the evolution of synthetic dyes and their applications in various industries. Methylene Blue was first synthesized by a German chemist named Heinrich Caro in the mid-19th century. This marked a significant milestone in the development of synthetic dyes, as it was one of the first synthetic dyes to be created.

One of the earliest and most notable applications of Methylene Blue was its use as a dye in the textile industry. Its vivid blue color made it a popular choice for dyeing fabrics, and it played a pivotal role in the transition from natural dyes to synthetic ones during the Industrial Revolution. This shift revolutionized the textile industry, leading to the production of more vibrant and colorfast fabrics.

In the realm of medicine, Methylene Blue gained prominence in the late 19th century as a treatment for various ailments. It was initially used as an antimalarial agent and later found applications in the treatment of methemoglobinemia, a condition where the oxygen-carrying capacity of blood is compromised. Over time, its medical uses expanded to include its role as a diagnostic tool, a staining agent in microscopy, and a treatment for certain psychiatric conditions.

1.3 Uses and Applications

Methylene Blue has a remarkably diverse range of uses and applications, making it a versatile compound with wide-reaching significance:

- **Medical Applications:** Methylene Blue is used in medicine for various purposes.

It serves as a medication to treat methemoglobinemia, a condition in which hemoglobin in the blood is unable to transport oxygen effectively. It also finds use in the management of cyanide poisoning and as an indicator dye in surgical procedures to assess blood flow.

- **Microscopy and Histology:** In biology and pathology, Methylene Blue is a valuable staining agent. It helps researchers and medical professionals visualize cells and tissues under a microscope. Its affinity for cellular structures makes it an essential tool for highlighting specific features within biological samples.

- **Psychiatric Treatment:**
  Methylene Blue has shown
  promise in the treatment of
  mood disorders such as
  depression and bipolar disorder.
  Research has explored its
  potential as an adjunctive
  therapy, although its
  mechanisms of action in this
  context are still under
  investigation.

- **Environmental Applications:**
  Methylene Blue is employed in
  environmental science for water
  quality testing. It can act as an
  indicator for redox reactions
  and has been used to assess the
  presence of pollutants and
  contaminants in water systems.

- **Textile and Industrial
  Dyeing:** Although less
  prominent today, Methylene

Blue is still used in the textile and paper industries as a dye. Its ability to impart a striking blue color to materials has historical significance in these fields.

- **Scientific Research:** Beyond its established applications, Methylene Blue continues to be a subject of scientific research. Its chemical properties and interactions with biological systems make it a valuable tool in various experimental studies.

Methylene Blue, with its vibrant color and multifaceted properties, has a long and storied history. From its origins as a synthetic dye, it has evolved into a versatile compound with significant implications in medicine, biology, and environmental science. Its continued use and exploration in various fields underscore its enduring importance in the modern world.

CHAPTER 2

Chemistry of Methylene Blue

2.1 Molecular Structure

The molecular structure of Methylene Blue (MB) is both fascinating and integral to its properties and functions. MB belongs to the phenothiazine class of compounds and consists of a complex aromatic ring system. Its molecular formula is $C_{16}H_{18}ClN_3S$, and its structural elements can be broken down as follows:

- **Aromatic Rings:** Methylene Blue contains three fused aromatic rings, making it an aromatic compound. These rings, composed of carbon and hydrogen atoms, contribute to its deep blue color and are responsible for its ability to absorb and emit specific wavelengths of light.

- **Heteroatoms:** Within the aromatic rings, there are two nitrogen atoms (N), one sulfur atom (S), and one chlorine atom (Cl). The nitrogen atoms are part of dimethylamino groups ($-N(CH_3)_2$), which play a crucial role in the compound's charge and interactions with other molecules.

- **Positive Charge:** Methylene Blue is a cationic dye, meaning it carries a positive charge. This positive charge is located on the nitrogen atoms of the dimethylamino groups. This charge allows MB to readily interact with negatively charged molecules, such as DNA, proteins, and cellular components, making it useful in various applications.

- **Methyl Groups:** The presence of two methyl ($-CH_3$) groups attached to each nitrogen atom further influences the molecule's charge distribution and reactivity.

- **Chlorine Atom:** The chlorine atom is attached to one of the aromatic rings and is responsible for the compound's chloride salt form, commonly used in various applications.

2.2 Chemical Properties

Methylene Blue exhibits several key chemical properties:

- **Water Solubility:** Methylene Blue is highly soluble in water, forming a stable aqueous solution. This property is essential for its use in various medical, biological, and staining applications.

- **Redox Properties:** One of the most remarkable chemical properties of Methylene Blue is its redox activity. It can readily undergo reversible redox reactions, transitioning between a reduced, colorless form (leucomethylene blue) and an oxidized, blue form. This property is exploited in various diagnostic and analytical applications, such as testing for redox potential in biological systems.

- **pH Sensitivity:** Methylene Blue's color and stability are pH-sensitive. The compound can change color or degrade under extreme pH conditions. This property is considered when using MB in various applications, especially in histology and microscopy.

2.3 How it Works

The versatile nature of Methylene Blue arises from its unique chemical structure and redox properties. Here's how it works in various contexts:

- **Medical Use:** In medicine, Methylene Blue is used to treat methemoglobinemia, a condition where hemoglobin is unable to carry oxygen efficiently. MB acts as a reducing agent, converting methemoglobin (a non-functional form of hemoglobin) back to its oxygen-carrying state (hemoglobin). This restoration of hemoglobin's functionality is vital for oxygen transport in the body.

- **Staining in Microscopy:** When used as a staining agent in microscopy, Methylene Blue is attracted to cellular components like DNA and acidic polysaccharides. It binds to these structures due to its cationic nature, allowing researchers to visualize and differentiate various cellular components and structures under a microscope.

- **Redox Indicator:** Methylene Blue serves as a redox indicator in various chemical and biological assays. Its color change from blue to colorless (when reduced) or vice versa (when oxidized) is used to monitor redox reactions and assess the redox potential of systems. This property is valuable in analytical chemistry and biochemistry.

- **Psychiatric Treatment:** Although the exact mechanisms are not fully understood, Methylene Blue has been explored for its potential antidepressant and mood-stabilizing effects. It may influence neurotransmitter systems and cellular metabolism, but further research is ongoing in this area.

Methylene Blue's molecular structure, chemical properties, and redox activity make it a versatile compound with applications in medicine, microscopy, chemistry, and potentially even psychiatry. Its ability to interact with and influence biological systems and redox reactions makes it a valuable tool in a range of scientific and medical contexts.

CHAPTER 3

Safety Precautions

3.1 Handling Methylene Blue Safely

Handling Methylene Blue (MB) safely is crucial to minimize potential risks and ensure your well-being. Here are some safety precautions to follow when working with MB:

- **Wear Personal Protective Equipment (PPE):** When handling MB, always wear appropriate personal protective equipment, including gloves, safety goggles, and a lab coat or protective clothing. This will help prevent skin contact and accidental splashes.

- **Work in a Well-Ventilated Area:** Ensure that you work in a well-ventilated area, such as a fume hood, to minimize exposure to MB fumes or aerosols. If proper ventilation is not available, consider wearing a mask or respirator as needed.

- **Avoid Ingestion and Inhalation:** MB should never be ingested, and inhaling its dust or vapor should be avoided. Be cautious when working with powdered forms of MB and ensure you don't create aerosols that can be inhaled.

- **Use Lab-Safe Handling Techniques:** Employ safe

laboratory techniques, such as using pipettes and containers specifically designated for MB, to prevent cross-contamination and ensure accurate measurements.

- **Prevent Spills and Splashes:** Be careful when transferring MB solutions to prevent spills and splashes. Use spill containment materials like absorbent pads or spill kits if necessary.

- **Wash Hands Thoroughly:** After handling MB, wash your hands thoroughly with soap and water, even if you wore gloves. Remove contaminated gloves carefully and dispose of them properly.

3.2 Storage Guidelines

Proper storage of Methylene Blue is essential to maintain its stability and prevent accidents. Here are some guidelines for storing MB safely:

- **Store in a Cool, Dark Place:** MB should be stored in a cool, dark place away from direct sunlight and heat sources. Exposure to light can degrade its color and efficacy.

- **Keep Containers Tightly Closed:** Ensure that containers holding MB are tightly closed when not in use. This prevents evaporation and minimizes the risk of spills.

- **Label Containers Clearly:** Clearly label all containers containing MB with its name, concentration, and any hazard warnings. This helps prevent confusion and accidental exposure.

- **Store Away from Incompatible Substances:** Keep MB away from incompatible chemicals, especially strong reducing agents or acids. Improper storage near incompatible substances can lead to hazardous reactions.

- **Follow Manufacturer's Recommendations:** Always follow the manufacturer's recommendations for storage conditions and shelf life, as these may vary depending on the form and purity of MB.

3.3 Potential Hazards

Methylene Blue is generally considered safe when handled properly, but there are potential hazards to be aware of:

- **Skin and Eye Irritation:** Contact with MB can cause skin and eye irritation. In case of contact, immediately rinse the affected area with copious amounts of water and seek medical attention if irritation persists.

- **Inhalation Risk:** Inhaling MB dust or vapor can irritate the respiratory system. Ensure good ventilation and use respiratory protection if working with concentrated forms of MB.

- **Potential Allergic Reactions:** Some individuals may be sensitive or allergic to MB. If you experience allergic reactions like skin rashes, difficulty breathing, or swelling, seek medical attention promptly.

- **Toxicity and Ingestion:** Ingesting MB can be toxic and should be avoided at all costs. In case of accidental ingestion, seek immediate medical help.

- **Environmental Impact:** MB can have adverse effects on aquatic environments. Proper disposal and wastewater treatment are essential to prevent environmental contamination.

By following these safety precautions and being aware of potential hazards, you can work with Methylene Blue safely and minimize the associated risks. Always refer to safety data sheets and guidelines provided by the manufacturer for specific information on handling and storage.

CHAPTER 4

Methylene Blue in Medicine

4.1 Medical Uses

Methylene Blue (MB) has several medical uses, primarily due to its unique properties as a redox-active compound. Here are some of its key medical applications:

Treatment of Methemoglobinemia: Methemoglobinemia is a condition in which hemoglobin loses its ability to transport oxygen efficiently. Methylene Blue is used as an antidote for this condition. When administered intravenously, MB acts as a reducing agent, converting methemoglobin back into functional hemoglobin. This helps restore the blood's oxygen-carrying capacity.

Treatment of Cyanide Poisoning: MB can also be employed in the treatment of cyanide poisoning. It works by facilitating the conversion of cyanide ions into less toxic substances, such as cyanate, through redox reactions. This helps counteract the toxic effects of cyanide.

Diagnostic Aid: In surgical and diagnostic procedures, MB can be used as a visual aid to assess blood flow. When injected into the bloodstream, it quickly distributes and colors the blood, allowing surgeons to visualize vessels, detect leaks, and assess tissue perfusion.

Potential Psychiatric Uses: While still under investigation, there is ongoing research exploring the use of

MB in psychiatry. Some studies suggest that MB may have potential as an adjunctive treatment for mood disorders such as depression and bipolar disorder, although more research is needed to establish its efficacy in this context.

4.2 Dosage and Administration

The dosage and administration of Methylene Blue vary depending on the specific medical condition being treated and the patient's age and weight. It is essential to follow medical guidance and prescription instructions closely. Here are some general guidelines:

- **Methemoglobinemia:** The typical intravenous dose for

methemoglobinemia in adults is 1 to 2 milligrams per kilogram (mg/kg) of body weight, administered slowly. The dosage may be repeated if necessary. In pediatric cases, the dosage may be lower, and it is administered under medical supervision.

- **Cyanide Poisoning:** Methylene Blue is administered intravenously at a dose of 1 to 2 mg/kg of body weight. This dose can be repeated as needed based on the severity of poisoning. It is usually given as part of a comprehensive treatment protocol for cyanide poisoning.

- **Diagnostic Use:** The dosage and administration for diagnostic purposes depend on the specific procedure and the patient's condition. It is typically administered intravenously, and the dose is determined by the medical team.

- **Psychiatric Use:** If MB is being investigated as an adjunctive therapy for mood disorders, the dosing and administration would be determined by a psychiatrist based on the individual patient's needs. This is an area of ongoing research, and dosing guidelines may evolve.

4.3 Side Effects and Risks

While Methylene Blue is generally safe when used as directed by medical professionals, it may be associated with some side effects and risks:

- **Local Skin Irritation:** When injected intravenously, some patients may experience local skin irritation or discomfort at the injection site.

- **Mild Nausea and Vomiting:** These side effects are rare but can occur, particularly at higher doses.

- **Serotonin Syndrome:** In rare cases, excessive use or high doses of MB may lead to serotonin syndrome, a potentially life-threatening condition characterized by symptoms such as agitation, confusion, rapid heart rate, and high body temperature. This risk is more significant when

MB is used with other serotonergic medications.

- **Allergic Reactions:** Although rare, allergic reactions to MB can occur. Symptoms may include skin rashes, itching, swelling, and difficulty breathing.

It is crucial to inform your healthcare provider about any pre-existing medical conditions and medications you are taking to ensure safe administration and to monitor for potential side effects during treatment.

4.4 Interactions with Medications

Methylene Blue can interact with various medications, potentially affecting their effectiveness or causing adverse reactions. Some important interactions to be aware of include:

- **Serotonergic Medications:** MB can interact with serotonergic drugs (e.g., selective serotonin reuptake inhibitors or SSRIs) and increase the risk of serotonin syndrome. Combining MB with these medications should be avoided or closely monitored by a healthcare professional.

- **MAO Inhibitors:** The combination of MB with monoamine oxidase inhibitors (MAOIs) can lead to severe hypertensive reactions. This combination should be avoided.

- **Antihypertensive Medications:** MB may

interfere with the action of antihypertensive medications, potentially leading to increased blood pressure.

- **Drugs Metabolized by CYP Enzymes:** MB can inhibit certain cytochrome P450 (CYP) enzymes in the liver, which may affect the metabolism and clearance of drugs that are substrates for these enzymes.

Before undergoing any treatment involving Methylene Blue, it is essential to provide your healthcare provider with a comprehensive list of all medications, supplements, and herbal remedies you are taking to ensure safe and effective treatment and to minimize the risk of drug interactions.

CHAPTER 5

Methylene Blue in Biology and Microscopy

5.1 Staining Techniques

Methylene Blue (MB) is widely used in biology and microscopy for its staining capabilities. Staining techniques with MB involve the application of MB solutions to biological samples to enhance contrast and reveal specific structures or components. Here are some common staining techniques:

- **Simple Staining:** In simple staining, a single stain like Methylene Blue is applied to a biological specimen. It uniformly colors all components of the cell, making it easier to visualize and study them under a microscope. This technique is often used to identify the basic morphology of cells and nuclei.

- **Differential Staining:** Methylene Blue can be part of differential staining methods like the Gram stain in bacteriology. In Gram staining, MB is used along with other stains to distinguish between different types of bacteria based on the characteristics of their cell walls. Gram-positive bacteria retain the stain and appear purple, while Gram-negative bacteria do not and appear pink.

- **Vital Staining:** Vital staining with MB involves using the dye on live cells to observe specific cellular functions or structures. For example, MB can be used to stain mitochondria or other organelles within living cells, allowing researchers to monitor cellular processes.

- **Histological Staining:** In histology, MB is commonly used to stain tissue sections for microscopic examination. Hematoxylin and eosin (H&E) staining, a widely used histological technique, often includes MB as part of the staining process to differentiate cell nuclei (stained by hematoxylin) and cytoplasm (stained by eosin).

5.2 Microscopic Applications

Methylene Blue has numerous applications in microscopy due to its staining properties and affinity for cellular components. Here are some key microscopic applications:

- **Cell Morphology:** Methylene Blue is frequently used to examine cell morphology and structures under a light microscope. It can highlight cell nuclei, cytoplasm, and other organelles, aiding in the identification and characterization of different cell types.

- **Microorganism Identification:** In microbiology, Methylene Blue staining helps identify and classify microorganisms. Gram staining, for example, differentiates bacteria into Gram-positive and Gram-negative groups, providing valuable information about their cell wall structure.

- **Mitochondrial Staining:** MB can be used to stain mitochondria within cells. This allows researchers to visualize the distribution and health of these essential organelles, which are involved in energy production.

- **Cytological Research:** Methylene Blue is used in cytological research to stain and analyze cellular samples, especially in studies involving cell cultures and cytospins. It aids in the visualization of cell morphology and intracellular structures.

5.3 Sample Preparation

Proper sample preparation is crucial when using Methylene Blue in microscopy to achieve accurate and clear results. Here are some steps involved in sample preparation:

- **Fixation:** Before staining, biological specimens need to be fixed to preserve their structure. Common fixatives include formaldehyde or ethanol. Fixation helps prevent degradation of cellular components and maintains the integrity of the sample.

- **Sectioning (for Tissues):** In histology, tissues are typically embedded in paraffin wax, sliced into thin sections using a microtome, and mounted on glass slides. These sections are then deparaffinized and rehydrated before staining with Methylene Blue.

- **Slide Preparation (for Microorganisms):** Microorganisms can be directly smeared onto microscope slides, air-dried, heat-fixed, and then stained with Methylene Blue. This method is commonly used for bacterial smears in Gram staining.

- **Staining Protocol:** Follow a standardized staining protocol, which includes the application of Methylene Blue solution to the sample for a specific duration. Rinse excess stain with distilled water, and if necessary, apply a counterstain to enhance contrast.

- **Mounting:** After staining, samples are usually covered with a glass coverslip using a mounting medium (e.g., glycerol or a resinous mounting medium) to prevent drying and protect the specimen during microscopy.

Proper sample preparation ensures that the stain is evenly distributed, and cellular structures are clearly visible under the microscope. It's essential to follow established protocols and adjust staining conditions based on the specific requirements of your microscopy study.

CHAPTER 6

Methylene Blue in Environmental Science

6.1 Water Quality Testing

Methylene Blue (MB) plays a crucial role in water quality testing and environmental monitoring. Its applications in this field include:

- **Redox Indicator:** MB is used as a redox indicator to assess the redox potential of water bodies. It undergoes a reversible color change from blue (oxidized form) to colorless (reduced form) depending on the prevailing redox conditions. This property allows environmental scientists to monitor the oxidative or reducing nature of water samples, which can provide insights into the presence of pollutants or changes in water quality.

- **Monitoring Organic Matter:** MB can be employed to detect and quantify the presence of organic matter in water. High levels of organic matter can be indicative of pollution or eutrophication (excessive nutrient content), which can impact aquatic ecosystems.

- **Determination of Oxygen Levels:** MB can be used to estimate the concentration of dissolved oxygen in water samples. It participates in redox reactions that are sensitive to the presence of oxygen, making it a useful tool in assessing the health of aquatic ecosystems.

6.2 Biological and Chemical Indicators

Methylene Blue serves as both a biological and chemical indicator in environmental science:

- **Biological Indicator:** In aquatic ecology, MB can be used to assess the metabolic activity of microorganisms and biological communities in water bodies. The reduction of MB by microorganisms is an indicator of their metabolic activity. Changes in the rate of MB reduction can signal shifts in microbial populations or the impact of pollutants on aquatic ecosystems.

- **Chemical Indicator:** As a chemical indicator, MB can reveal the presence of various contaminants in water. For example, it can react with sulfides, which may be present in water as a result of pollution or natural processes. The formation of a blue precipitate indicates the presence of sulfides.

6.3 Environmental Impact

While Methylene Blue is valuable in environmental science applications, it's important to consider its environmental impact:

- **Toxicity to Aquatic Life:** Methylene Blue, when released into water bodies in significant quantities, can be toxic to aquatic organisms. Therefore, it should be used with care and in controlled amounts in environmental monitoring.

- **Environmental Persistence:** MB can persist in aquatic environments, potentially affecting the water chemistry and ecosystems over time. Proper disposal and management are essential to mitigate any long-term environmental impact.

- **Use in Environmental Remediation:** On a positive note, MB has been explored as a tool for environmental remediation. Its ability to interact with contaminants and pollutants can be harnessed in processes like wastewater treatment and the removal of heavy metals from water.

Methylene Blue plays a significant role in environmental science by serving as a versatile indicator for assessing water quality, monitoring biological activity, and detecting contaminants. However, its potential environmental impact underscores the importance of responsible usage and disposal practices when working with this compound in environmental monitoring and research.

CHAPTER 7

DIY Experiments with Methylene Blue

7.1 Creating a Methylene Blue Solution

Before conducting DIY experiments with Methylene Blue (MB), you'll need to create a suitable MB solution. Here's a basic guide to creating an MB solution:

Materials Needed:

- Methylene Blue powder or crystals (available from scientific suppliers)

- Distilled water

- A glass container (such as a beaker or glass jar)

- Stirring rod or glass pipette

Procedure:

1. Measure the amount of MB powder or crystals you need for your experiment. The specific amount will depend on your experiment's requirements.

2. Place the MB powder or crystals into the glass container.

3. Add distilled water to the container. The amount of water should be sufficient to dissolve the MB completely. The

concentration of the MB solution will depend on your experiment, so measure the water volume accordingly.

4. Stir the mixture using a stirring rod or glass pipette until the MB is completely dissolved. This may take some time, so be patient.

5. Once the MB is dissolved, you have created your Methylene Blue solution. Label the container with the solution's concentration and store it in a safe location, away from direct sunlight and heat.

7.2 Simple Experiments for Beginners

Here are a couple of simple experiments you can conduct using Methylene Blue:

Experiment 1: Redox Reaction with Vitamin C

Materials Needed:

- Methylene Blue solution
- Vitamin C (ascorbic acid) tablets or powder
- Clear glass or plastic cups
- Water

Procedure:

1. Prepare two clear cups with equal amounts of water.

2. In one cup, add a few drops of Methylene Blue solution and mix it to create a blue-colored solution.

3. Crush a Vitamin C tablet (or use Vitamin C powder) and add it to the second cup of water. Stir until the Vitamin C is dissolved.

4. Pour the blue Methylene Blue solution into the cup with the dissolved Vitamin C.

5. Observe the color change. Methylene Blue will be reduced by the Vitamin C, turning colorless or pale.

Experiment 2: Methylene Blue as a pH Indicator

Materials Needed:

- Methylene Blue solution

- Vinegar (acidic) and baking soda (basic)

- Clear glass or plastic cups

- Water

Procedure:

1. Fill two cups with water.

2. In one cup, add a few drops of Methylene Blue solution and mix it to create a blue-colored solution.

3. In the other cup, add a small amount of vinegar to make it acidic. In another container, mix water and baking soda to make a basic solution.

4. Carefully add drops of the acidic vinegar solution to the blue Methylene Blue solution. You'll notice a color change

from blue to green or colorless as the pH becomes more acidic.

5. Repeat the process with the basic baking soda solution. You'll observe a color change back to blue as the pH becomes more basic.

7.3 Safety Guidelines for Experiments

When conducting experiments with Methylene Blue or any chemical, safety should be a top priority. Here are some safety guidelines to follow:

- **Wear appropriate protective gear:** Depending on the experiment, wear safety goggles, gloves, and a lab coat or apron to protect your eyes, hands, and clothing.

- **Work in a well-ventilated area:** Ensure good ventilation to prevent inhaling any fumes or aerosols that may be produced during the experiments.

- **Use small quantities:** Work with small amounts of chemicals to minimize risks and waste.

- **Dispose of waste properly:** Dispose of any leftover solutions and materials according to local regulations. Methylene Blue should not be poured down the drain without proper treatment.

- **Keep emergency supplies handy:** Have access to safety equipment like an eyewash station and a chemical spill kit in case of accidents.

- **Follow instructions:** Always follow experiment instructions precisely, and do not deviate from recommended procedures or concentrations.

- **Never ingest chemicals:** Under no circumstances should you ingest any chemicals used in experiments, including Methylene Blue.

Following these safety guidelines and conducting experiments in a responsible manner, you can enjoy educational and informative experiences while minimizing risks.

CHAPTER 8

Future Trends

8.1 Future Trends and Developments

The use of Methylene Blue (MB) in various fields continues to evolve, and several future trends and developments are likely to emerge:

1. **Advanced Medical Applications:** Research into the medical applications of MB is ongoing. Future developments may include the refinement of MB-based therapies for conditions such as depression, bipolar disorder, and neurodegenerative diseases. Additionally, innovative drug delivery systems using MB as a carrier could enhance its efficacy and reduce side effects.

2. **Nanotechnology and MB:** Nanotechnology holds promise for enhancing the properties and applications of MB. Nanoformulations of MB may improve drug delivery, increase its stability, and enhance its specificity for targeting specific tissues or cells. This could lead

to more effective treatments and diagnostics.

3. **Environmental Monitoring:** The importance of water quality and environmental monitoring is growing, driven by increasing concerns about pollution and climate change. MB's role as a redox indicator and its ability to detect pollutants may lead to the development of more advanced and sensitive monitoring techniques for assessing environmental health.

4. **Green Chemistry and Sustainability:** The synthesis and use of MB may evolve to become more environmentally friendly. Research into greener synthesis methods and sustainable production practices

could reduce the environmental footprint associated with MB manufacturing.

5. **Combination Therapies:** MB's potential as an adjunctive therapy in psychiatry and other medical fields may lead to the exploration of combination therapies. Researchers may investigate how MB interacts with other drugs or treatment modalities to enhance therapeutic outcomes.

6. **Biotechnology and MB:** Advances in biotechnology may enable the development of novel MB-based bioprobes and biosensors. These could be used for real-time monitoring of biochemical processes within living cells or as

diagnostic tools for various diseases.

7. **Public Awareness and Education:** As the accessibility of scientific information increases, there may be a growing interest in DIY experiments and citizen science projects involving MB. Public education and awareness efforts will likely be important to ensure safe and responsible experimentation.

8. **Regulatory Considerations:** With the expanding use of MB in medical and environmental applications, regulatory agencies may revisit guidelines and regulations related to its production, use, and disposal to ensure safety and environmental protection.

9. **Interdisciplinary Research:** Collaborations between researchers from different disciplines, such as chemistry, biology, medicine, and environmental science, will continue to drive innovation in MB's applications. These collaborations may lead to the discovery of new uses and optimization of existing ones.

It's essential to stay informed about these trends and developments, as they can have a significant impact on the utilization of Methylene Blue in various fields. Researchers, healthcare professionals, and environmental scientists will continue to explore the full potential of MB while addressing safety, ethical, and environmental considerations.

CHAPTER 9

Beyond the Basics

9.1. Methylene Blue in Analytical Chemistry

Analytical chemistry is a field dedicated to determining the composition, structure, and properties of substances. Methylene blue, with its versatile properties, has found a significant place in analytical chemistry, contributing to a wide range of analytical techniques and methods. Here are some advanced applications of methylene blue in this domain:

Redox Indicator

Methylene blue serves as an excellent redox indicator in analytical chemistry. Its characteristic color change from blue to colorless, corresponding to its reduction from the oxidized (blue) to the reduced (colorless) form, is valuable in titration experiments. This property allows researchers to determine the concentration of reducing agents in a sample, which is crucial in various chemical analyses.

Electrochemistry

In electrochemical studies, methylene blue is frequently used as a redox-active compound. It can undergo reversible redox reactions on the surface of electrodes, making it a suitable candidate for constructing electrochemical sensors and biosensors. These sensors can detect specific analytes, such as biomolecules or ions, with high sensitivity and selectivity.

Spectrophotometry

Methylene blue's absorption spectra exhibit distinct peaks at different wavelengths depending on its oxidation state. This property is exploited in spectrophotometric measurements. Researchers can quantify the concentration of methylene blue or the substances it interacts with by analyzing the changes in absorption spectra, a technique often used in the analysis of pharmaceuticals and complex chemical mixtures.

Complexation Studies

Methylene blue can form complexes with various ions and molecules, including DNA and RNA. This property has applications in studying molecular interactions and binding affinities. In analytical chemistry, researchers employ methylene blue to investigate the binding characteristics of molecules, aiding in drug discovery and biomolecular research.

www.ingramcontent.com/pod-product-compliance
Lightning Source LLC
Chambersburg PA
CBHW062246290526
45794CB00006B/2426